KEVIN BROWN

Hiking for Beginners

First published by Woven Brink Publishing LLC 2024

First edition

This book was professionally typeset on Reedsy.
Find out more at reedsy.com

Contents

Introduction

So you're interested in hiking, huh? Well, guess what? I love hiking, and I'm thrilled to share my knowledge and experiences with you. My name is Kevin Brown, and I enjoy hiking on different kinds of trails in different environments. So why should you listen to me? Because I, too, started as a beginner hiker and didn't know which way was up. Through my experiences hiking, I've found what works and what doesn't. I've hiked in many national parks, state parks, and local trails.

Hiking is more than just a walk in the woods—it's an adventure that can transform your life. We've all heard that hiking and being in nature is good for your physical and mental health, relaxing, and clearing your head. But there's so much more to it than that. Hiking is something you can do by yourself, with a friend, or with a group. And it can be free! Whether you're scaling mountain peaks or strolling through a local park, hiking offers endless opportunities for discovery and personal growth.

As a beginner, you may be excited about getting into hiking and nervous about what you may be getting yourself into. These are all normal feelings. This book will help put your mind at ease by guiding you through everything you need to know to start your hiking journey. From selecting the proper clothing and gear to finding the perfect trail and mastering trail safety and etiquette, this book has got you covered.

I'm not here to tell you the history of hiking or tell you tales of traveling all over the world to find the perfect trail. This book is designed to help you find local trails in your area, no matter where you are, and prepare you for your first hike or second, whatever the case may be. My goal is to make hiking accessible, enjoyable, and safe for everyone, especially beginners.

So, lace up those boots, grab your backpack, and let's embark on this exciting journey together. The trails are calling, and incredible adventures await. I'll see you out there, ready to discover the beauty of the great outdoors!

Chapter 1: Getting Started

Why hike, you ask? Aside from the numerous health benefits, hiking is a fantastic way to escape the hustle and bustle of everyday life, even if only for an hour or so. It's a low-impact exercise that offers a surprising number of health benefits. Hiking is excellent for your cardiovascular system, easy on the knees, and strengthens all the muscles in your legs, feet, and ankles. It helps improve balance, boosts your immune system, and enhances endurance.

But the benefits of hiking extend far beyond the physical. I've dealt with mental health challenges, and I've found that being out in nature is the best way to settle down and clear my head. It's cheaper and far more exciting than going to a counselor. I've hiked in forests, mountains, and now I hike in the Southern Utah deserts. Each hike brings its own experiences and challenges, and every trail offers a new adventure.

Types of Hiking

Before you hit the trails, it's essential to understand the different types of hiking. Here are the main categories:

Day Hikes: These are perfect for beginners. They can be

completed in a day or less and require minimal planning and equipment. These are the kinds of hikes you'll want to start with. Don't think of it as a day hike; these can be completed in any amount of time.

Multi-Day Hikes: Avoid these when starting. They require overnight camping, permits, and a lot more gear.

Thru-Hiking: These long-distance hikes, like the Pacific Crest Trail, can last for months and involve significant planning. They're not for beginners but are something to aspire to as you gain more experience.

Choosing Your First Hike

Finding the right trail for your first hike is crucial. One excellent resource is an app called AllTrails, which I highly recommend. It's free to use, with a paid version offering additional features. The free version provides plenty of information to find, navigate, and track your hike. It's what I use, and I love it. You might be wondering, "What if there's no cell phone reception?" Great question! You can download the maps of the trail you plan to hike before venturing out. This enables you to use the app without reception—keep that battery charged!

It's very important to start with a trail that isn't too difficult. This will help you ease into hiking without scaring you off. What determines a hike's difficulty level? Factors include length, terrain, altitude, weather, trail condition, etc. Hiking trails are generally not paved; you'll be walking on dirt, sand, rocks, and sometimes crossing streams. The AllTrails app can inform you about these conditions. User reviews and pictures provide additional insights before you embark on your hike.

Hiking in the mountains with tall trees around you is very different from hiking in the desert with no shade. Know what you're getting into. We've all heard stories of people getting lost, suffering heat strokes/exhaustion, or worse. These can all be prevented by being prepared and using common sense.

Set Realistic Goals

You don't have to summit Mt. Everest on your first hike. Just find a local trail near your house and hike it for about 20 minutes. Start small. If you're exhausted, head back and recover. The next time you go hiking, try to go just a little further.

Remember, the key to enjoying hiking is setting realistic goals, choosing the right type of hike for your ability, and starting small. Hiking is meant to be enjoyable and fulfilling, not overwhelming or discouraging.

Let's remember the benefits of hiking: physical health, mental well-being, and the joy of exploring nature. By choosing the right type of hike for your ability and starting small, you'll set yourself up for success. In the next chapter, we'll dive into the essential gear you'll want to consider to make your hikes safe and comfortable. Stay tuned, and let's get ready to gear up!

Chapter 2: Essential Gear

As my dad always says, "He who packs light does not have what he needs." When it comes to hiking, this couldn't be more accurate. Even on short hikes, things can get dangerous quickly if you're not prepared. Let's dive into the essential gear you'll need to make your hiking experience safe and enjoyable.

Boots

Boots are arguably the most important piece of gear you'll invest in. Comfort here can make or break your hike. You want them snug but not too tight. There are several different types of hiking shoes to consider:

Hiking Shoes: Lightweight and flexible, these are great for shorter hikes. These are excellent starter shoes for hiking.

Hiking Boots: I use Merrell Moab hiking boots. They provide extra support for my ankles and are fantastic for longer hikes and varied terrain. I've hiked in Yosemite National Park and the extreme deserts of Southern Utah in these boots, and they've been fantastic. Also great for crossing low streams as they're waterproof.

Backpacking Boots: These are more for thru-hiking as they offer more support and durability. I don't have experience with these since I don't go for multi-day hikes.

Any sporting goods store around you will have a great selection of footwear you can try on. The main thing is comfort. I've found that I like to go about a half-size up from my regular shoes so my toes have more room to move without jamming them into the front of the shoe when going downhill.

And don't forget about socks! Socks are just as crucial as boots when it comes to preventing blisters. I used to wear regular cotton socks, which led to sweaty feet and blisters, especially in the desert. Now I wear wool socks, which are much more comfortable, help prevent blisters, and don't stain from the dirt. Carrying a blister kit in your backpack is also a good idea.

Clothing

Have you ever heard the expression, "The weather is only as bad as the clothes you have on"? It's true. When hiking, you'll want to consider wearing layers, as the temperature and your body's cooling system can change rapidly. The harder you're working, the hotter you'll get. Think of a base layer, mid layer, and outer layer. Avoid Cotton. I repeat, avoid cotton. Cotton retains moisture and doesn't dry quickly, leading to blisters, chafing, and even hypothermia. Instead, opt for moisture-wicking materials.

Depending on the type of hike you're doing, you may want to consider a pair of lightweight pants to avoid brushing up against vegetation and prevent bug bites. However, if it's a heavily trafficked trail, shorts are generally perfectly fine.

Backpacks and Tools

There are packs of different sizes, but for beginners, a smaller pack with hydration is a great place to start. I use a CamelBak MULE, which I love. It has a 3L water reservoir, plenty of room for a jacket, snacks, essential tools, and easy access to things I might need regularly. It's designed with ventilation, so it doesn't sit flush against my back, which I appreciate. When looking for a pack, I highly recommend this option.

When it comes to backpacks, comfort is key. Head over to a sporting goods store and try them on. For beginner hikes, you don't need anything too expensive or crazy. Remember, we're starting at 20 minutes.

My first significant hike taught me a real lesson. My friend and I were hiking from Glacier Point to Vernal Falls in Yosemite—about 8-9 miles. When we got to Vernal Falls, I was almost out of water. With the refill station out of order, this became a serious issue. We still had to get back. My friend shared his water with me, but I was also out of food. It was hot, I was tired, and my entire body was sore. By the time we finished, my body went into shock. I couldn't stop shaking; I was hot and cold at the same time. It was miserable. What should have been an enjoyable hike turned scary simply because I wasn't prepared. I didn't make the same mistake two days later when we went on an even longer hike from Yosemite Valley up to Half Dome. I was prepared for that one!

Navigation Tools

Packing a map is a good idea, but they're useless if you're like me and don't know how to read them. I rely on GPS. Download the map of the hike you're planning beforehand, bring a battery charger bank, and you're good to go. A compass can also be handy.

First Aid and Safety

I once went on a hike and brushed my leg against a plant with a stick poking out. Nothing crazy, just a simple plant with a simple stick. That stick opened up my leg, and I couldn't stop bleeding. It didn't hurt, but it was making a mess. Now I travel with a small first aid kit: antiseptic wipes, bandages, and blister treatment. Although hiking at night isn't recommended when you're first starting, it's never a bad idea to carry a headlamp with you. It's a light that attaches around your head.

Bringing a multi-tool or knife is also helpful. And don't forget sunscreen and a hat, depending on the weather. If you're someone who doesn't have the best balance, trekking poles can help out immensely. Again, any decent sporting goods store will have many options to choose from.

Packing Tips

When packing your gear, remember that placing heavier items lower in your backpack will help keep you balanced. Putting heavier items on top squishes your gear and can make you fall backward.

By investing in the right gear and being prepared, you'll set yourself up for a successful and enjoyable hiking experience. Now that you're equipped with the knowledge of essential gear, let's move on to planning your hike!

Chapter 3: Planning Your Hike

Now that you've got your gear all sorted out, it's time to start planning a hike! Finding a suitable hike near your location can be an exciting part of the adventure. There are many resources available to help you discover trails, such as the Internet, apps, social media sites, and even just asking fellow hikers.

Discovering Trails

One of the best ways I discover new hikes is by using an app called AllTrails. This app is a treasure trove of hiking information and features. It can give you directions from wherever you are to the trailhead's parking lot (the trailhead is the starting point). Not only does it direct you to the exact location of where you should park, but it also provides step-by-step directions for the hiking route. If you veer off course, the app will let you know. This app has all kinds of maps, elevation profiles, timing, and safety features.

Instead of promoting the app, I'll simply say to download it and play around with it. Even if you're technically challenged, I believe you can figure it out. It's pretty straightforward and user-friendly. AllTrails is just one of many hiking apps available, but it's my go-to because of its comprehensive database and ease of use.

Basic Trail Etiquette and Tips

Now that you've found the perfect beginner hike to start with, let's go over some basics to ensure a smooth and enjoyable experience:

Parking: Not all trailheads have designated parking lots. Sometimes, you might park on the street in a residential neighborhood. Don't be alarmed by this; just make sure you're not blocking driveways or parking in restricted areas.

Parking Fees: Some trails require a parking fee. There will usually be clear instructions on how to pay when you arrive. It's a good idea to have some cash or a credit card handy.

Permits: Certain trails require permits, especially in more popular or protected areas. Check ahead of time whether you need a permit and how to obtain one.

Trailhead Signs: Always read the signs at the trailhead. They provide helpful information, including maps, trail lengths, difficulty levels, and any specific rules or warnings for the area.

Leave No Trace: This is crucial. Pack out what you pack in. Leave the trail as beautiful as you found it, if not better. This means carrying all your trash with you and not disturbing the natural environment.

Understanding Different Hiking Areas

When trying to find a hike, it's important to know whether you're headed into a national park, state park, or another public land. Each type of land has its own set of rules and regulations:

National Parks: Include famous places like Yosemite, Zion, and Bryce. They are often well-maintained and have many resources for hikers, but they can also be crowded. National parks usually require an entrance fee.

State Parks: Examples include Snow Canyon, Quail Creek, and Sand Hollow. State parks are great alternatives to national parks and can offer equally stunning scenery with potentially fewer crowds. They may also require an entrance fee or a state park pass.

Public Land: Bureau of Land Management (BLM) These are your local trails. I went on a hike and the trailhead was literally between two homes on a residential street. These types of hikes generally don't have any amenities such as restrooms or water stations.

Planning Your Hike

Planning your hike involves more than just picking a trail. Here are some additional tips to help you prepare:

Research the Trail: Look up reviews, photos, and maps of the trail. This can give you an idea of what to expect regarding scenery, difficulty, and potential hazards.

Check the Weather: Always check the weather forecast for the day of your hike. Weather can change quickly, especially in mountainous areas, so it's important to be prepared for anything.

Trail Conditions: Vary greatly depending on the season and recent weather. Mud, snow, or fallen trees can make a trail more challenging. The AllTrails app often includes recent reviews from other hikers about the current trail conditions.

Plan Your Route: Decide how far you want to hike and plan your route accordingly. Make note of any landmarks or points of interest along the way.

Time of Day: Consider the time of day you'll be hiking. Morning hikes can be cooler and less crowded, while afternoon hikes might offer more warmth and daylight. Always allow enough time to complete your hike before dark; but have a headlamp just in case.

Emergency Plan: Have a plan in case something goes wrong. Know the location of the nearest hospital or ranger station and let someone know your hiking plans, including your expected return time and the route you're taking.

Planning a hike is part of the adventure. By taking the time to research and prepare, you'll ensure a safe and enjoyable experience. Now that you're equipped with the knowledge to find and plan your hike, let's get ready to hit the trails and explore the great outdoors!

Chapter 4: Preparing for the Hike

Proper preparation is key to ensuring a safe and enjoyable hike. This chapter will guide you through the steps to get ready for your hike, from physical conditioning to packing your gear and understanding safety precautions. Being well-prepared will enhance your hiking experience and keep you safe and comfortable on the trail.

Physical Conditioning

Building up your physical strength and endurance is important before heading out on your first hike. Start with simple activities like walking, jogging, cycling, or swimming. These exercises will help condition your body for the physical demands of hiking. You don't have to do anything too taxing, but it's essential to get your body moving and accustomed to regular exercise.

I'm an avid runner, I strength train three times a week, and I ride my bike once or twice a week. Even with all this activity, when I go out for my first hike of the year, my shins are sore for a couple of days. The next hike I do, I'm fine. Even for people who are in shape, going on the first hike will make you sore.

Don't let this discourage you from going again. The more you do it, the easier it gets.

Walking around your neighborhood or at a park with your gear on is also a good idea to get comfortable and familiar with it. There's nothing more annoying than trying to remember which pocket in your backpack you put something in while you're hiking. Test all your gear out. Make sure your boots aren't rubbing your feet in the wrong way. Ensure the backpack is comfortable and does not rub against anything. Gradually increase your distance each time. Try going up and down stairs; this will help with hiking up hills.

Packing for Your Hike

When packing for your hike, remember to include the following essentials:

Water: Hydration is key. Bring enough water for the duration of your hike and more.

Food: Pack high-energy snacks like trail mix (ever wonder where the name comes from?), nuts, dried fruit, or energy bars.

Navigation Tools: Bring a map, compass, or GPS device. Download the map of the hike beforehand if using an app.

First-Aid Kit: Carry basic first-aid supplies, including antiseptic wipes, bandages, and blister treatment. Hand sanitizer is not a good option for treating a cut; trust me!

Multi-Tool or Knife: Handy for a variety of situations.

Sun Protection: Sunscreen, a hat, and sunglasses are essential, especially in open or high-altitude areas.

Extra Clothing: Layer up. Bring a lightweight jacket or rain gear in case the weather changes.

Trekking poles: Helpful for stability and balance, especially on uneven terrain.

Camera or binoculars: For capturing the beauty of nature.

Insect repellent: To keep bugs at bay.

Headlamp.

Safety Precautions

Safety should always be a top priority when hiking. Here are some key safety tips to keep in mind:

Tell someone where you're going: Share your hike route with someone and let them know when you expect to return. Even if it's an easy hike, get used to letting someone know your plans. Have check-in times and a plan for what to do if you don't check-in. These simple steps can save your life if you get lost or injured.

Have a plan B: If the weather changes or the hike becomes too difficult, turn around. It's better to live and hike another day. If you start to feel exhausted, turn around. Don't try to push yourself too far.

Be aware of elevation changes: When you start a hike, you're likely at a lower elevation than where you'll end up. Weather can change dramatically depending on the time of year and your location. Just because it's nice and sunny when you start doesn't mean it'll be nice and sunny at your turnaround point.

Wildlife and Plant Awareness and Safety

Understanding the wildlife and plants you might encounter on your hike is important for your safety:

Wildlife: Research the wildlife you might encounter and understand their behaviors. Sometimes this information is listed on signage at the trailhead. For example, in Yosemite, I encountered bears; while in Southern Utah, I see tortoises and lizards. Be cautious of the creatures you might encounter, as you're in their habitat.

Plants: Most actively used trails are clearly marked and have enough foot traffic to keep the plants at bay. However, sometimes you might want to get a closer look at something and not realize you just rubbed up against poison ivy. Be aware of what you're walking on. Thorns are not much fun, either!

Preparation is the foundation of a successful hike. By building your physical fitness, packing wisely, and taking safety precautions, you'll be ready to tackle the trails confidently. Remember to stay flexible and adaptable, as conditions can change quickly in the outdoors. With thorough preparation, you'll be set for a safe and enjoyable hiking adventure. Now it's time to get on the trail!

Chapter 5: On the Trail

Now that you've prepared thoroughly for your hike, it's time to hit the trail. This chapter will guide you through essential hiking techniques, trail etiquette, staying hydrated and nourished, and managing common issues that may arise during your hike.

Hiking Techniques

Start slow and build up. Pace yourself. This is not a competition. Enjoy the views and take it all in. Look down to avoid obstacles; look around and enjoy nature and the wildlife. Stand up tall to prevent your backpack from causing you to lean forward and hunch. Don't forget to breathe! When going uphill, take shorter steps and slow down. When going downhill, watch your footing and remain in control.

Trail Etiquette

Yield to hikers going uphill. They have a more strenuous climb, and maintaining their momentum is very important. If you pass someone, make your presence known. If you're on a dirt trail, they may be able to hear you coming if they're not engaged in music or conversation. It doesn't hurt to say passing on your left or right. You might even strike up a conversation.

I was hiking much faster than a woman up ahead of me. She asked me if I was familiar with the trails around here. I said yes, and long story short; we hiked the entire 5.25 miles together. Come to find out, she lived not too far from where I used to live. You never know who you will meet on the trails, so it pays to be friendly with everyone. Say hi. Even if they don't say hi back, keep saying hi to people. You may find yourself running into the same people again.

Step off the trail to let faster hikers, groups, mountain bikers, or horses pass. Yes, you might find mountain bikers and horses with you! Bringing your dog to hike with you is perfectly acceptable if they're on a leash. Remember to pick up after them. Try not to stomp on the vegetation and stay on marked trails.

When going for a hike, try to keep the noise levels down. You can talk, but screaming kids and loud music make it less enjoyable for others. People go on hikes to enjoy nature and its calm and quietness.

Staying Hydrated and Nourished

When you start hiking, you may not need to worry too much about water purification. When you start going on longer, more remote hikes, you'll want to consider that. For this book for beginners, I'm not going to get into that. A water bottle or water reservoir in your backpack is enough. A Gatorade or other drink with sugar and electrolytes is also a very good idea. If it's too hot out and you're sweating, your body loses salt. You can replenish this with an electrolyte drink or salty snacks.

I went on a hike with my mom, and even though she kept telling me she was okay, by the time we were about 100 yards from the car, she was in heat exhaustion. She had to lay down and get more fluids in her right away. The lesson we both learned is don't try to be tough. It's difficult to get out of heat exhaustion. You feel lightheaded, dizzy, and very uncomfortable. The best thing is to avoid it completely by staying hydrated and nourished. If you're getting tired, turn around and tell your group that you cannot continue. Keep drinking, and if you need to use the restroom, well, find a tree or a bush. Some trailheads have restrooms, the AllTrails app will tell you if they're available or not.

It's a good idea to bring trail mix, nuts, dried fruit, chips, crackers, and even protein bars. These can hold up well in a variety of different weather conditions and will give you enough energy to keep going. As I have found out the hard way, protein bars can melt, so choose wisely which ones to bring.

Managing Common Issues

Blisters, scratches, and minor injuries are normal things that can come with hiking.

Blisters and Minor Injuries:

Preventing Blisters: Wear moisture-wicking socks and well-fitted boots. Use blister prevention tape or moleskin on hot spots before they become blisters.

Treating Blisters: If you get a blister, stop and treat it promptly. Clean the area, apply a blister pad or moleskin, and cover with a bandage. This should be in your hiking backpack.

First-Aid for Injuries: Carry a basic first-aid kit with bandages, antiseptic wipes, pain relievers, and any personal medications. Know how to treat common injuries like cuts, scrapes, and sprains.

Fatigue and Motivation:

Take Breaks: Rest periodically to avoid overexertion. Find a scenic spot to take a break, hydrate, and have a snack. Take some pictures.

Stay Positive: Keep a positive attitude, even when the trail gets tough. Focus on the beauty around you and the sense of accomplishment you'll feel.

Set Small Goals: Break the hike into manageable segments and celebrate reaching each milestone.

Navigating Difficult Terrain:

Uphill Sections: Use a steady, rhythmic pace and lean slightly forward. Take shorter steps and use trekking poles for added support.

Downhill Sections: Bend your knees slightly and take shorter, controlled steps. Use trekking poles to help maintain balance and reduce impact on your knees.

Rocky or Uneven Terrain: Watch your footing carefully and use your trekking poles for stability. Take your time to navigate challenging sections safely.

Conclusion

Congratulations on completing this guide to hiking for beginners! You've embarked on a journey that not only takes you through breathtaking landscapes but also enriches your physical and mental well-being. Hiking offers a unique blend of adventure, tranquility, and personal growth, and you are now equipped with the knowledge and skills to fully embrace this rewarding activity.

Throughout this book, we've explored the essential aspects of hiking, from understanding the types of hikes and choosing the right gear to planning your adventures and mastering trail etiquette. Each chapter has provided you with practical advice, insights, and tips to ensure that your hiking experiences are safe, enjoyable, and fulfilling.

Recap of Key Points

Getting Started: We delved into the various types of hikes and the many benefits of hiking, helping you understand why this activity is so popular and beneficial to your health.

Essential Gear: We covered the critical gear needed for hiking, emphasizing the importance of proper footwear, clothing, backpacks, and other tools.

Planning Your Hike: This chapter highlighted the importance of research, understanding trail difficulty, checking weather conditions, and adhering to regulations to ensure a successful hike.

Preparing for the Hike: We discussed physical conditioning, smart packing, and safety precautions, laying the groundwork for a well-prepared adventure.

On the Trail: This chapter offered practical hiking techniques, trail etiquette, tips for staying hydrated and nourished, and ways to manage common issues, ensuring you are ready to tackle the trail confidently.

Hiking is more than just reaching a destination; it's about appreciating the journey, immersing yourself in nature, and finding joy in every step. Each hike offers new experiences, challenges, and opportunities to learn and grow. As you continue to explore different trails and terrains, you'll discover more about yourself and the world around you.

Remember, every hiker started as a beginner. With each hike, you'll gain more confidence, skill, and appreciation for the natural beauty surrounding you. Stay curious, stay safe, and always respect the environment and fellow hikers.

Your hiking journey doesn't end with this book. Countless trails are waiting to be explored, each with unique beauty and challenges. Consider joining hiking groups, participating in outdoor workshops, or even setting ambitious goals like completing a long-distance trail. The possibilities are endless, and the hiking community is always welcoming and supportive.

As you lace up your boots and head out on your next adventure, take a moment to reflect on how far you've come. Enjoy the serenity of the wilderness, the thrill of discovery, and the satisfaction of pushing your limits. Hiking is a lifelong journey filled with endless adventures and unforgettable moments.

Thank you for allowing me to be part of your hiking journey. I hope this guide has provided you with valuable insights and the confidence to explore the great outdoors. Now, it's time to hit the trails and create your own hiking stories.

If you found this book helpful, I would really appreciate an honest review to help others like you discover the benefits of hiking. It would mean a lot!

Happy hiking!

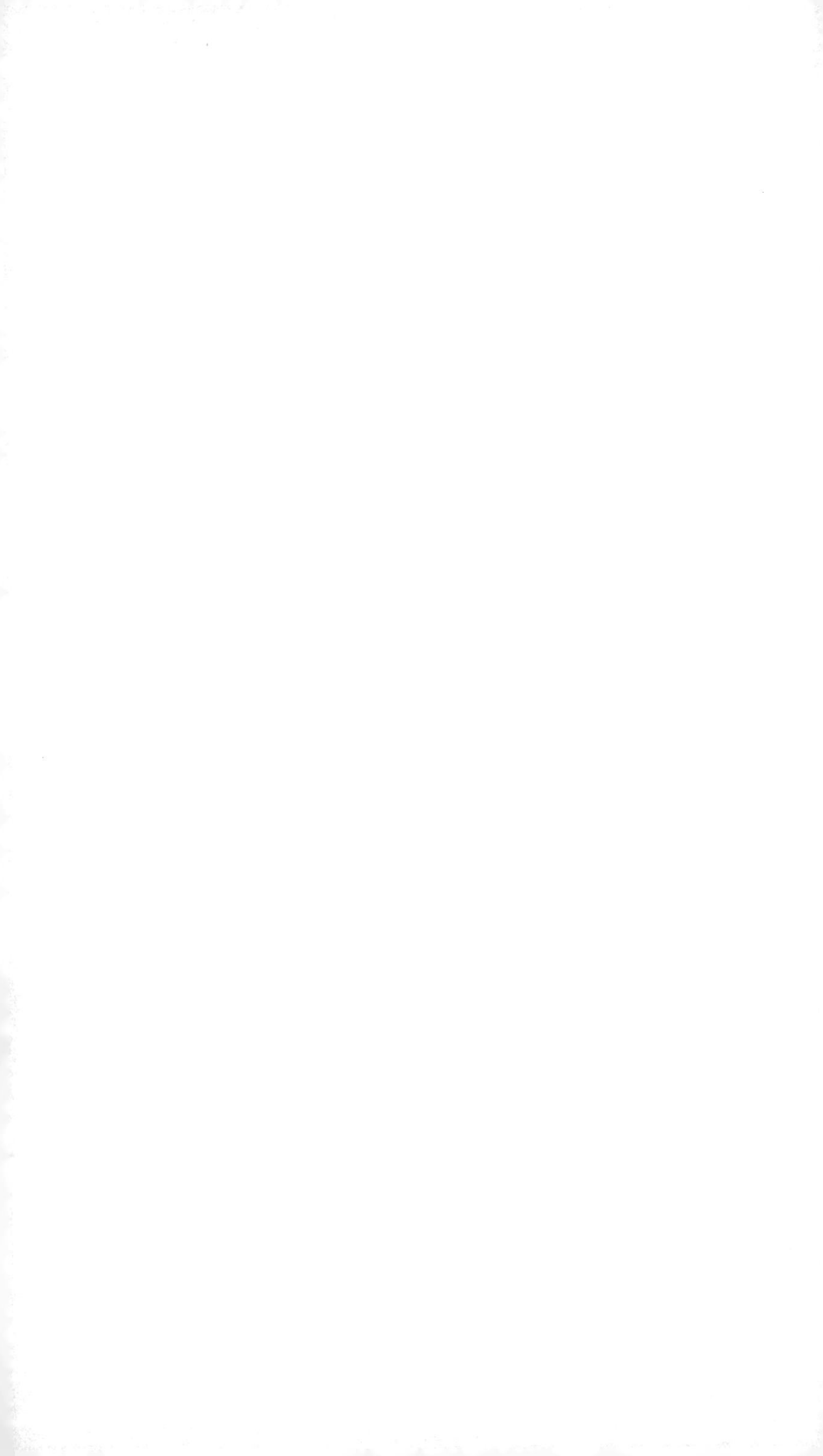

www.ingramcontent.com/pod-product-compliance
Lightning Source LLC
Chambersburg PA
CBHW051239250726
48656CB00003B/1030

9798328243049